CONTENTS

INTRODUCTION

T his is the book I wish I had read when life was all about migraines, pain, anxiety and survival. I had tried all the medications and treatments that healthcare had to offer. Nothing helped and I did not want to live anymore. If I had read this book then, it would have given me hope for life and a direction forward when I no longer knew what to do with myself. I would have avoided detours, lost time and a strong feeling of loneliness.

Amongst other things, this book is about what helped me to no longer be afraid of living my life. To despite migraines, live a life I didn´t think was possible, a life full of joy, love and creativity. A life where I can do whatever I want; work, exercise, travel, enjoy life, meet friends, create, evolve, discover and learn new things.

I won´t make any promises of you becoming migraine-free, but with an open mind and a willingness to explore other ways to look at migraines and pain, I want you to feel hopeful of having a wonderful and fantastic life despite migraines.

For 25 years I suffered from migraines up to 20-25 days a month. Most of those days the pain was so terrible I ended up spending a lot of my time in dark rooms together with nausea and anxiety. It took courage, determination and self-love to let go of control and face the unknown. I finally decided that I actually wanted to participate in my life, and not just survive in a dark room. To choose life, quality of life, was the most important decision to make. I needed courage to go my own way. If I had listened to everyone who told me that there is nothing more to do, you have to live like this, you have to accept your situation, you will not be able to work etc., I would not be sitting here today. I needed self-love not to give up, to continue to encourage myself that I am valuable and in fact worthy of a fantastic life. To believe in myself when no one else did. That migraines are not my fault, but that I have a responsibility for what I do with my life. Having a migraine is not a punishment from hell for doing something wrong. I also needed self-love to understand that I don´t have to achieve anything to be valuable, I don´t have to compare myself with anyone else and I don´t have to prove anything to anyone.

Today, when I look back on my life and what I have learnt so far from living with migraines, I feel gratitude. Migraine is a serious illness, but it also puts things at the forefront, we have to actively choose joy and life over suffering, otherwise the risk is that time just passes by and we miss out on all our dreams. When I finally realised that pain does not at all have to mean suffering, the door to freedom was opened. When I realised that all my suffering was something I did to myself, the realisation also came that I had a choice. I can´t control my migraine, but I can decide for myself whether to choose the suffering, or the joy and love for life. Since the day I actively chose joy and love, my life turned for the better. Of course, I have highs and lows like everyone else, but nowadays I know that it´s temporary and that it passes. I have opened the door to freedom and now there is no turning back.

During the years when I fumbled my way to better health and living, I at first felt extremely lonely, but I eventually found people who supported me. By support I don´t mean those who wanted me to see "the reality", that migraines never go away and that I have to accept the pain, but the people who surrounded me in different ways and who through their attitude and love taught me that everything is possible. They taught me what acceptance really is, that I am not defined by my illness and that I can have the life I want.

THE STARTING POINT OF THE BOOK

This book is written from the bottom of my heart, with love and compassion for all who suffer from migraines. It´s written with the greatest understanding of what it´s like to be affected by migraines. I know how it is. I know what it´s like to lie in the dark, literally, but also in a darkness of hopelessness and despair. I know what it's like to feel completely powerless. I know what it's like to wake up in the morning and long for the evening when you can return to bed again. I know what it's like to be in so much pain that you believe something is going to break inside your head. I know how it feels when you think you´re going to die, because you can´t endure such pain and nausea. I know how it feels when you want to die because it feels like you have no life. I know what it´s like to be depressed, to have anxiety and feel guilty. I know what it's like to have mood swings and blame everything and everyone, then regret it bitterly. I know what it's like to meet incompetent healthcare professionals. I know what it´s like to sit and cry at the health centre week after week with a doctor who thinks you should just drink a glass of wine and relax. I know how it feels to take so much medicine that you have to be detoxified. I know what it's like not to be believed in. I know what it's like to feel alone in the world. I know what it's like to cry every single day and worry about your children and the future. I know what it's like to think you've done something wrong and migraines are the punishment from hell. I know how it feels when the days go by and you don´t have the strength to participate. I know what it's like when all the loved ones meet and have fun and you can´t take part. I know what it's like to be in a dark room on Christmas Eve. I know what it's like to have children and be annoyed and not be able to listen because my head hurts. I know what it's like to feel guilty. I know what it´s like to try and make an effort to have a better life but nothing helps.

I also know what it's like to get out of the dark and start walking towards the light. I know that when I didn´t give up on being worthy of a great life, the insights finally came. I know there are two steps forward and one back. I also know that if I can, so can you. I also know that if we help each other, it's easier. I know that who we are beneath all the layers of illness and pain can be brought out. I know we can find happiness, enjoyment and lust for life despite migraines. I know life is amazing. I know that love from fellow human beings can hold us up when we´re in doubt. I also know that despite the hell migraines can bring, it can also be a turning point if we find the courage to take the step. I know we need to surround ourselves with positive forces that provides energy. I know that in order to have a better life, we must be prepared to change and evolve. And above all, I know that we are not our achievements and that we are not selfish when we take care of ourselves, on the contrary, when we get energy and feel better, we have the ability to spread joy wherever we go.

I also know that if we continue to do what we have done so far, the result will be the same as what we experience every day. To change a habitual pattern is always difficult, no matter what. It's even harder when your head hurts, but the rewards are even greater when we do.

TRIGGERS

A trigger is something that´s often discussed when it comes to migraines. It´s usually various foods that cause migraines, the weather, hormones, stress and everything else between heaven and earth, and the advice from both healthcare and well-meaning fellow human beings is often to avoid your triggers and accept your limitations. If I had followed the advice to avoid my triggers and accept my limitations, I wouldn´t have recovered at all. When I felt my worst, the migraines were triggered from pretty much everything. I woke up with migraines every single morning and the only way forward was to challenge my triggers two steps forward and one back. At the same time, it´s important to remember that this doesn´t mean that we should simply just go on and do everything we feel like doing without stopping. It means that we need to become aware of our triggers and acquire strategies on how we handle them. We have to challenge ourselves in a way that makes it possible to succeed, which means patience, confidence that things will get better and courage to let go of control.

Triggers from certain foods and beverages are common in many people. Refraining from foods and beverages that trigger migraines does not have to be a limitation in itself. There are endless of recipes to discover fantastic food that gives us the nutrition and energy our body needs. A lot of triggers are from unhealthy foods and additives that are not good for anyone. The problem is often about changing a habit and phasing out unhealthy food without giving up, even if it doesn´t have an immediate noticeable effect on the migraine. Eating healthy becomes a piece of the puzzle for better health. Triggers from certain foods and drinks can also be about expectations from others, that we should eat what they offer, drink some alcohol with dinner and not bother with wanting other alternatives. Additionally, it´s not uncommon for food and sweets to become an addiction, when our mood sways we often comfort eat to stun our emotions instead of facing them.

A common trigger for migraines is internal stress where a major contributing factor is our negative thoughts. Our negative thoughts are camouflaged as different things, but the bottom line is about loving oneself, feeling valuable and having a good self-esteem. It´s about us all being worthy of a happy and fulfilling life, and we should *allow* ourselves to live life in full. Most of us know that all people are equally worth, that we are valuable whoever we are and that we are not defined by our achievements or the roles we take on throughout life. We also know that our differences are the contrasts that enriches us and help us grow. We all have our experiences and baggage to handle and challenge, and the inner stress it causes gives different symptoms to different people. When we don´t allow ourselves to live the life we deep down want and long for, everyone is somehow reminded of this through physical and / or mental symptoms. Because we are social beings, we want to fit in and we often adapt to the external framework that tells us how we should be, what we should do and what we should not do. We listen to others around us more than we listen to our inner selves, we compare ourselves to others, which often means that we go against or even crush our own dreams and desires. Our longing is suppressed, and when we start feeling bad as a result, we blame ourselves for not being good enough, we convince ourselves that there is something wrong with us because we can´t feel happy and satisfied, and we feel that we have to make an even bigger effort to fit in and to be like everyone else.

Performance anxiety is a major contributing factor to internal stress. We have to do something, be active, achieve, otherwise we are lazy, incompetent and unsuccessful, or something else that evokes a feeling of not being good enough as we are. We live in a society where achievement is seen as strength and success. Many of us also grew up receiving praise and attention, many times all in goodwill for what we have accomplished and because it´s a virtue to make an effort. But what happens to us if we no longer can work or achieve things? Who are we if we can´t work or, in our own eyes, contribute something to others?

Performance anxiety becomes a challenge for us who suffers from migraines. It´s often difficult, if not impossible, to achieve things with an aching head and nausea. We get ourselves down because we don´t have the strength / ability to perform, we feel worthless, we develop a bad conscience and everything becomes worse, the inner stress becomes more prominent. We strive to perform, we work even though we don´t have the strength, we take care of others even though we don´t have the strength, we do one thing or another even though we don´t have the strength. And the migraine becomes increasingly worse, the tension in the body is growing and the inner struggle becomes harder. The thoughts of what we should do, what we should have done but didn´t do and how unsuccessful we are wears us down. Performance anxiety can also affect us in our aim to feel better and appear when we make more of an effort to feel better. We try more medications and treatment methods, we try to exercise more and to avoid more, eat better and explore new discoveries. It often doesn´t lead to more energy or less pain, but we simply go around in circles and we can´t get out.

Since we´ve learnt that hard work is what´s required to achieve success, it can be difficult to see that the solution may be to reduce performance requirements, and also drop them completely in certain contexts, so we simply stop making an effort instead. Learning to reduce certain performance requirements and completely let go of others can be a big challenge, but we can start with small steps, put an end to everyday life and think about what we really "have" to do and why. For whom do we have to achieve something? What happens if we ease our own demands? Many times, it´s our own demands that are the most considerable, the people around us often have no issues with us going a bit easier on ourselves.

To *compare* ourselves to others is also about doubting ourselves and our worth. Each and every one of us is completely unique with different backgrounds and internal and external prerequisites. In whatever way we compare ourselves to others, it evokes inner stress because it doesn´t go hand in hand with the fact that we are worthy just as we are. If we compare ourselves to others, we will diminish ourselves by, for example, noticing that we are on sick leave when others work and earn money. We barely have the energy walk around the house when others are exercising and running. We have to lie in a dark room when others go on excursions. If we compare ourselves to others and come to the conclusion that we are "better" than them, we also diminish ourselves because such a statement means that we must be or do something special to be good enough. None of this makes us feel better.

When we encounter someone who has succeeded in something that we
ourselves long for or dream of, we can feel jealousy and irritation, which is
expressed in negative thoughts and possibly negative expressions towards the
other. This is never about the other person, but this is about us seeing and
being reminded of where we are in relation to our dreams and our longing.
We often look for excuses and explanations to why we find ourselves where
we are, and why we have not come any further, which evokes a sense of
failure as we put focus on the limitations.

It´s only when we *don´t have to* compare ourselves to others that we can
relax. When we accept ourselves the way we are and where we are at the
moment in life, we become filled with energy. When we can honestly and
genuinely congratulate others, who have achieved what we also wish for
ourselves, we focus on what we want in the future instead of retaining a sense
of failure. We feel hopeful and get filled with more energy because we put
focus on the possibilities.

If, instead of comparing ourselves to others, we see other people as teachers
and inspirers, we can encourage ourselves to stick to our intentions to feel
better in the long run. There are many people who have come out of very
difficult situations in life and who are willing to share some fantastic life
experiences and lessons. If we allow ourselves to be inspired and rejoice in
how these people have succeeded, we feel hopeful that we too can succeed. If
we help each other and share our successes, we get filled with energy.

To please others and to care about what other people think is rooted in the
fear of not being accepted and liked by others, and with this I don´t mean we
shouldn´t help out or show consideration for others in a friendly, equal and
healthy way. What creates an inner stress is when we try to adapt to others in
a way that doesn´t match who we are or what we want. We adapt to social
interactions, cultures and unwritten rules on how to act and behave together
with others because we don´t want to stand out and do something that´s
considered strange or different. We easily hold ourselves back, and we are
more concerned of other people´s wellbeing instead of making room for
ourselves. Many of us don´t say what we´re actually thinking, and instead
keep our needs and desires to ourselves. We are there for others and do things

that we might not actually want to do. We don´t set boundaries and let fear rule, we please and care more about what other people think than of our own wellbeing.

When we please and / or care about what others think in a way that limits us, we notice it by having energy taken away from us. Sometimes it´s very clear that we go against our own needs, but we don´t want to acknowledge it because it feels difficult to say no and make someone else disappointed or angry. We sometimes even get a migraine before we do something, because we deep down do not want to. We´re being told by the migraine that this is not okay. The question is, what´s most important, to please others or to feel good?

If we practice not judging, criticise or to compare ourselves or others, it becomes easier to accept ourselves and others just as we are, equals. When we know our own worth, we don´t need the approval of others to feel okay, just as others don´t need our approval for them to feel okay. When we know our own worth, we can set boundaries and maintain our integrity. Other people's criticism, judgment or negative opinion is not about us. It´s about people who can´t handle their own problems and who instead blame others for their own internal struggles. Sometimes we might need feedback from others in order to evolve, which is very different, because constructive feedback is not about deciding on another person´s worth.

As we begin to change in our ambition to feel better, we'll encounter challenges. We have to show more courage and love and respect ourselves enough not to fall back when our surroundings begin to react. People in general don´t like change and when we start taking more responsibility for our lives and set boundaries, it is more difficult for our surroundings to control and influence us. Some people may react by trying to hold us back or convince us that what we are doing is simply not a good idea. Somehow, they are threatened or afraid of how our decisions will come to affect them. It can involve family members, but it can also apply to care staff. We may well be considered tricky of difficult, because we don´t do what´s expected. It´s important to remember that this is not about us. People who truly genuinely want us to recover will encourage us to take our own responsibility and trust that we ourselves know what is best for us. They will cheer us on, rejoice in every step of the way and be of great support.

Guilt and shame take an enormous amount of energy and are the root to a lot suffering. The difference between guilt and shame is that shame is about "I am wrong", while guilt is about "I have done wrong". In essence, there is a reason for us to feeling guilt and shame because it shows that we can distinguish right from wrong.

It´s not uncommon for us who have migraines to often feel guilty about things we aren´t in control of, things we could not have known about or things we have chosen in good faith. To feel guilty, we have to be able to take responsibility, but we can´t take responsibility for other people or circumstances. We can´t take responsibility for things that happened that we could not or can not control. As long as we carry guilt, we carry tensions in the body that causes symptoms that often lead to migraines or tension headaches. Some feelings of guilt are deep, and we may sometimes need professional help to deal with them, while others are often about us making unreasonable demands on ourselves. We must learn to forgive ourselves, not for the things we couldn´t control, because we forget that we are valuable and do our best based on what we know and can do. If we act on the basis of good intentions without judging, criticising, comparing and evaluating, we can state that we have done our best based on current circumstances. If we act consciously, we have nothing to regret afterwards and we can minimise the feelings of guilt.

So, what does it mean if we feel guilty because we have migraines? Does it mean we could have done something different? If we feel guilty because we have a migraine, it basically means that we are responsible for the cause of it. We are only to blame for what we have done with the intention of harming others or ourselves and therefore feeling guilty for migraines would mean that we caused migraines to, for example, avoid work, avoid taking care of our children or avoid going out and meeting friends. This sounds unlikely to say the least, so what it is about? In my opinion, there are two options in answer to that question. Either we are not honest with ourselves in the sense that we haven´t taken care of ourselves, we have ignored the signals from our body and heart and ignored our own needs, which we know makes us feel worse. When we then have to cancel, we know deep down that it could have been different. Alternative number two is that we have chosen the victim position. For some reason, we don´t take responsibility for things being the way they are. I don´t mean that we are sick, we don´t have that control, but we don´t respect or love ourselves enough to take responsibility for our needs. Instead, we hurt ourselves with self-blame and negative thoughts. A good way to avoid feeling guilty for migraines is that we take responsibility *before* we end up in a situation that can evoke those feelings. Most likely, there are many of us who sometimes choose to do the things we know has a high risk of resulting in a migraine as a consequence. If we take responsibility for the consequences, there is no reason to feel guilty. In these cases, we can, for example, ask ourselves "I am aware that this can contribute to a migraine tomorrow (when I already have something planned). Am I willing to take the consequences without blaming myself? Will I think this choice is okay tomorrow?"

Worry - worrying about the next attack is a stress trigger that many people recognise. All worry affects us in a negative way, it´s not just the worry for the next attack. We probably all know that worrying about different things takes energy and contributes to us not being able to feel good in the moment, even though what we are worried about has not happened. Many of the things we worry about never happen, but some worries become self-fulfilling prophecies, and migraine attacks are usually included in that category. In other words, we get migraines more often when we worry about getting it. Because worry is about something that may happen at a later time, we have no power whatsoever to do something about it, because we can´t control the future. When we worry, we miss what is happening here and now right in this moment, and in a way, it becomes like a resistance to the life that´s ongoing. As long as we worry about getting migraine attacks, or whatever it is that we are worried about, we let fear control our lives. When we focus on being in the now, being present in the moment, it means that we take back the power and authority over our lives. We can´t reach into the future and influence it, but what we create here and now can change where we end up tomorrow. If we create a calm here in this moment, enjoy it, immerse yourself in the feeling of just feeling good and appreciate what we have around us right now, we can´t worry about anything in the future at the same time. If we work on accepting the present just as it is, we have great opportunities to break the negative thought patterns, and consequently, the vicious circle. There are several good techniques to deal with worry and to focus on here and now. Mindfulness and meditation are well known and very effective. I have personal experience of moving forward in my life when fear and worry ruled for many years. It took 2-3 months of daily meditation to release a lot of the anxiety I have carried for years, and when the anxiety now appears, I know what to do. Letting go of worries and what we can´t control, and instead have confidence in life, is a very effective migraine medicine.

Becoming aware of what happens when we´re stressed and what impact it has, not only on the body, but also on an emotional level, is an essential for understanding ourselves better, having patience and being able to more easily reverse the downward spiral that we often have ended up in. When we become aware of how stress contributes to our thoughts being limited, and how it in turn can be difficult for us to see opportunities and solutions, we understand how important it is that we learn how to manage our everyday life and relax. When we learn to relax, both our body and mind, we activate the relaxation response. The more we activate it, the greater access we get to positive and creative emotions such as gratitude, love, joy, inspiration, power etc. Positive emotions help us to have more energy, which in turn helps us to look more positively at our own ability to influence our health.

When the relaxation response is activated, the level of stress hormones decreases, and the parasympathetic nervous system is activated. It´s only in this rested, relaxed state that the body can heal itself.

THE SUFFERING

Talking about suffering can be a sensitive chapter. In my opinion one of the reasons for this is that you confuse being a victim of / affected by an event with feeling like a victim. Anyone can be affected by tragedies, diseases and crime, and there are many people who are affected by war, torture, starvation and natural disasters. Suffering from something we have no control over induces both physical and mental reactions, and the feeling of powerlessness and fear can be overwhelming. These are completely natural reactions and people can suffer severely under these circumstances. The problems arise when the crisis is over and there is no longer an acute danger, and at the same time you hold on to your suffering by getting caught up in negative thought patters. We are held hostage by our own mind through an eternal negative cycle of thoughts about how powerless we are, about guilt and shame, about self-loathing and about how worthless we really are, that we are punished for something we have done "wrong", that our suffering is due to other people's faults etc. This happens over and over again, and if we don´t try to break the pattern, we get stuck in self-pity and nothing ever changes for the better. Sometimes professional help can be absolutely crucial to process trauma and difficult life events, and the help that everyone needs can vary based on the actual event and individual needs.

To stop thinking like we are the victim, we need to become aware of our behavior and thought patterns, and then decide that we want to make a change. This means that many things in life can change, including how our surroundings sees us, reacts and treats us. It can mean changes we need to be prepared to carry out when we decide to take responsibility for our lives. There are no shortcuts to feeling better or having the life we want. Choosing to take responsibility is the only solution, and to do this continuously.

Choosing the victim role means that we give away our power and authority over our lives to people and circumstances around us. If you are a victim, it means that it´s the circumstances that control, and when circumstances or people control our lives, the risk that we become like a feather in the wind is great, depending on what´s going on around on. Let's say we feel good when people understand us, are kind and positive, and we feel bad if someone is angry at us, rejects us or in other ways express themselves negatively and incomprehensibly. We feel good when the bus arrives as scheduled because we´ll then be on time and arrive when we planned to. But when the bus is delayed, we become stressed, irritated and in turn feel unwell. This means that we must try to control the circumstances, and it might work within the family, as our closest ones show consideration and do everything necessary for us to feel good, but in the rest of the world this is completely meaningless. There are people and circumstances everywhere who don´t do as we please. If we let circumstances and other people control how we feel, we always lose, we give away our own power of action. In fact, no one can make us feel bad if we ourselves don´t allow it through our own negative thoughts that have convinced us that we are powerless. Having a migraine is a difficult circumstance, but it doesn´t automatically mean that we have to feel bad emotionally. We are not powerless, on the contrary, we have more power in us than many know.

Getting caught up in the victim role is treacherous. It feels good when we get attention and comfort, people show consideration and take care of us. We may have friends or belong to a group that gives our suffering attention, and we feel safe and seen there. The problem is that we are digging a hole that´s getting harder and harder to get out of. Anger, jealousy, condemnation, self-destructiveness and other negative expressions are given free rein and it may even be that we, among our friends and other groups of people, come to the conclusion that we have a common enemy and we thereby confirm the injustices of life. The only thing this leads to is that all energy run out and we don´t feel any better, on the contrary, even more internal stress is activated which eats away at the body.

When we wait for the miracle medicine, the cure, the solution to our mood, we find ourselves in the victim role because it´s something beyond ourselves, a circumstance that will make us healthy and happy. I don´t mean that you shouldn´t take medicine that helps, what I mean is that once the medicine is here it may not work as well as we thought it would, or maybe the effect subsides after a while and then we start feeling bad again. When we take active responsibility for our well-being regardless of the circumstances, a miracle cure does not become crucial to our quality of life.

I think we all choose to play the victim role at regular intervals and it´s not something we should complain about, on the contrary, we have to be kind to ourselves and realise that we all do our best based on our experiences and our current life situation. The most important thing is that we learn to recognise the signs of when we are heading towards the victim position and immediately change direction.

Something that has helped me a lot that I can warmly recommend is to take part in other people's stories and in this way gain perspective. It´s easy for us to paint a pitch-black picture of our lives if we are lonely with our thoughts, or if we meet or in other ways have contact with other victims who confirm that picture. We can´t compare suffering, but what we can be inspired by is how other people have gone through very difficult life traumas and illnesses and are happy and grateful for life.

RELATIONSHIPS

One of the areas in life where the minds impact on the body is the greatest, is our relationships. Love doesn´t only heal the soul, but also the body. Loneliness, anger and bitterness are like poison to the body. A healthy relationship strengthens the relaxation response in the body. An unhealthy relationship activates the stress response.

To really think about what relationships we have and who gives and takes energy is crucial to how we feel. Being forced to spend time with people who in some way, consciously or unconsciously, try to control us or in another way influence who we are, contributes to inner stress and a feeling that we´re not worthy just as we are. It can be about a partner, family members, friends, colleagues, etc. The relationships that give energy and allow us to be ourselves, the relationships where we feel support, encouragement and freedom, are the relationships we must nurture.

To feel good in our relationships, we must set boundaries and stand up for ourselves. We must opt out of the relationships that puts us in the victim role or in another way contribute to destructive thoughts and feelings. Of course, it´s not easy, we are many times dependent on people around us and change evoke fear of being alone. It can also regard fear of not getting help when we are sick and etc.

The first step is to become aware of which relationships are not good for us and start there. Making small changes, starting to set boundaries and practicing relating to others in a way that prevents other people's negative energy from destroying us, causes us to slowly phase them out.

For me, the world of yoga has made the importance of relationships so clear.

Yoga has led me to people and opportunities that I would never have found in all the stress and activities. I have found new communities in my life full of people who give love, joy and acceptance, where we don´t compete, judge, compare or have opinions about one or the other. We wish each other the very best. We take responsibility for our lives. We choose to see the positives in other people, we laugh a lot, we look beyond the surface and attitudes. We are not defined by our illness, our age, our gender or our roles, we are valuable just as we are. We don´t have to explain ourselves to anyone because we don´t need anyone else's approval to be ourselves. We see our difficulties as challenges and hold each other extra tight when life is turbulent. These moments create a being that means creativity and one's own positive power can emerge. A context that provides positive energy, evokes relaxation and flow, and where tension and pain are absent. To me, these contexts contribute to a meaningful and happy life.

WORK

For us with migraines and other severe headaches, coping with a job can be a challenge. With chronic migraine, it can really feel hopeless, but even if the migraine appears less often, the very fear of having an attack can take a lot of energy. A very important part of our lives is what we do for a living, therefore it´s extremely important to us, just like for anyone, to really enjoy our work and feel that we´re in the right place to do what we are passionate about, to get stimulation and satisfaction. Employers have a vast responsibility for their staff, and a good boss works hard to create an environment that is surrounded by a minimal amount of stress.

There are several things we can do ourselves to influence the situation in our workplace. Firstly, it is extremely important that we enjoy our work. If we´re not happy with our work tasks or our colleagues, we´ll suffer even greater difficulties in coping with a functioning working life. Secondly, we need to keep track of our rights and obligations so that the starting point is ready for us. It´s always important to know where to begin. When this becomes clear, we get to the next step, which is what we personally need. Common to us who suffer from migraines is the need to work in a, as much as possible, stress-free a work environment. We may need adapted work tools depending on our task assignments, with the aim of reducing the risk of tension and strain on the body. Some people may need to work part-time or otherwise have their working hours adjusted. In other words, we need to start by making sure that the external circumstances are as favorable as possible.

When the external conditions become clear, we get to the part of work that only we ourselves can take responsibility for, namely our attitude and our ability to handle the stress that the job causes. It's about how we handle the situation if there is a lot or little to do, how we relate to our colleagues in day-to-day work, but also in relation to the fact that we may be absent from time to time. We need to take responsibility for having enough energy to work and for how we take care of ourselves, both physically and mentally, to feel good enough to cope with work. If we don´t learn to deal with stress and the approach towards our surroundings, it doesn´t matter how well-adapted our work conditions are. If we think about it, this is noticed when we´re on sick leave and may have the opportunity to rest and recover for several weeks or months without the stress we experience at work, but when it's time to return to work we are soon getting back into old habits, and soon the thoughts that we can´t do our job are back and the migraine arrives like a letter in the post.

It´s important to not let the migraine control our choice of work. If we do, it´s easy for us to end up where we don´t thrive (because we limit ourselves when we let migraine control) and when we don´t thrive, an internal stress with consequences is induced, such as migraine. The body and the heart strive for balance, and this also applies to mental well-being. This means that we´ll receive continuous signals that this is not what we want, signals in the form of negative emotions that lead to pain. At the same time, we have to be realistic and not run ourselves down with performance anxiety and fear of what others might think.

The time we live in is fantastic in the way that more and more jobs become flexible. There are opportunities to work from home or in other ways control your work, and there are many opportunities to thrive and make money despite migraines. The most important thing is to not limit your thinking but to think freely and then gradually start looking at what´s possible right now and start from there. There are many examples of people who have ended up not being able to work as they intended due to illness or other circumstances, but who, thanks to being forced to rethink, have found a new, even better meaning in their work. I myself have been a social worker for almost 30 years, and that is where my heart belongs. After working my way to total exhaustion to help others, I have now, after a few years, found an inspiring path with great opportunities that I probably never would have found if I had continued to move forward on the path I was on. Therefore, I am grateful that I was forced to listen to my heart in the end, even though it didn´t feel that way when I was right in the middle of all the chaos. Not feeling comfortable or ending up on sick leave due to stress can also, when we start feeling a bit

better and calm our thoughts, mean new opportunities and paths to
meaningful employment pursue.

CONTROL OR CREATE

Trying to control the circumstances (to control how we feel) means that we have to be allowed to hold on to the thing we want control over, so we know where it´s at. To resist, to fight to keep the circumstance in place, can claim all our energy.

What´s worst of all, is that having control is an illusion, at least the control that means getting circumstances and other people to behave in a certain way for us to allow ourselves to feel good. The more we try to control the circumstances, the more stiff, rigid and stringent we become. If we don´t look up, we end up straight down in the victim role, and then we lose strength and power to do differently.

However, we can train ourselves to control the approach to our surroundings, which means taking control of our mind and thoughts, and by that, in the long run, our emotions and reactions. It´s an exercise, just like training the muscles, which needs to be done continuously throughout life, but which gets easier and easier with time. If we stop exercising, we lose focus and it´s easy for us to fall back into old patterns. When we practice our inner control, we can make the decision on how to react (as opposed to just reacting), which reduces emotional storms and tensions. We become calmer and more stable, more confident in ourselves and are less often dragged down by feelings of guilt, because we think before we act and by that reduce the risk of us reacting to others. Internal control does not mean that we don´t care, on the contrary, we care about how we feel, we are kinder to ourselves and we project a calm energy, a calm and secure impression to our surroundings. In turn, this has a ripple effect and we support other people in a completely different way than otherwise. We make better decisions and trust ourselves. Practicing inner control requires self-awareness, responsibility and courage, because it means staying in the present together with the emotions that awakes in the moment, instead of disappearing into anxiety, the mind frame of a victim or other expressions of fear and powerlessness.

To assent to our creativity is a powerful way to evolve and release the flow and energy that heals us. When we find ways to express our creativity, we are filled with energy and soon find our balance again. When we open up for creation, we open up to the flow of energy that we need to make a change, and grasp the things we need to feel better, which happens when creation requires us to focus here and now. It´s in the present that we make the changes we need, it´s in the present that all our strength and power exist because we can neither reach into the past and change anything that has been, nor stretch into the future and change anything there. If we make time to create and challenge ourselves in a way we enjoy and fills us with energy, it will become easier to lessen the need for control. We challenge ourselves and at the same time think about why certain things really have to be a certain way. What is the purpose of this? We need to question and move the boundaries of our comfort zone bit by bit. Then we'll grow as human beings and let new opportunities into our lives.

Control and create are two opposites. When we put time and energy into controlling, we miss the opportunities that constantly appear in the moment. By focusing on control, we get caught up in the same old ways of thinking, which guarantees that nothing changes. We can´t expect to feel better if we continue to control and have the same thoughts we´ve had so far. If we look at our lives, we see the result from years of the same thoughts and patterns over and over again. And this will continue into the future if we don´t choose differently. When we let go of what we can´t control and let creativity in, anything can happen. We leave room for new ideas and we have the courage to try new things and an open mind for new opportunities. If we let go of control we have the courage to do more because we don't feel the need to control the result. If it goes well that´s great, if not then at least we have tried, and so, we move on. Letting go of control is really what we need in order to reduce the triggers we have that concern inner stress.

WHAT DOES GOOD HEALTH MEAN, TO BECOME WELL?

I t´s very important to really think about what it means to be healthy. We are all different and have different desires and frames of reference, but the absence of migraines does not automatically mean that we are healthy and well. When I felt my worst, I could after all sometimes experience a headache-free day and I appreciated that a lot, but I was still tired, exhausted and unfocused. I used to take the opportunity to do some extra activities those days which resulted in severe attacks the next few days. I told myself for a long time that my migraine had to go away in order for me to feel healthy. When I started thinking about what healthy meant to me, I came to the conclusion that it´s to feel joy, vitality, energy, to be creative and focused, have a clear brain and a strong body.

Most of us have at some point been advised by medical staff or by people in our surroundings to keep a migraine diary. In it you should write down how many attacks you have, what degree of difficulty it has and what medications you have taken. Some diaries also imply that you have to write down tension headaches. In addition to this, you should focus on your triggers and what triggered the attack. The point is to have grounds when you see your doctor and discuss which treatment would be suitable. I always think it's good to try being as concrete as possible when describing things to others, especially something as important as health. On the other hand, the question of what will happen if we focus too much on our migraine diary arises. Since it´s a diary, it means that we should put focus on it every day, then we can see what the weeks look like, and then the months and years. I kept a migraine diary for a long time, and it was not a fun read because according to my own logic I was healthy when I was headache free. It felt pretty hopeless because I had headaches and migraines pretty much everyday day year after year.

A few years ago, I had enough of my migraine diary. I decided to reverse the reasoning and stop keeping track of which days I had migraines, I really didn´t feel better about it. I started applying another strategy which means that when you want to quit something (in this case to focus on the number of days with migraines) you have to focus on what you want instead. It´s never a good strategy to remove something first, everyone that tried to stop something unwanted knows that just removing something does not automatically mean that the void that arises is filled with something good.

So, the strategy that works is *first* putting focus on what to fill the upcoming void with, and *then* stop. For the most part, we don´t even have to stop, the unwanted is phased out without much effort. In this case, it meant that I started turning the reasoning around and keeping a feel-good diary where I (even today) write down everything that makes me feel good, everything good I do for my health, what I am grateful for, and that allows me to continue to feel good and be happy. There is no focus on migraines. It´s a completely different feeling and energy to read the diary and see all the positive factors that actually exist every day and to praise myself when I see how many good things I do for my health. Try writing a success diary where you pay attention to all the positive things you do for yourself and take notes of how your body feels.

LISTEN TO THE BODY

A starting point for feeling better that we can´t skip, is that we love and take good care of our bodies. To dislike, or even hate one's body (or a body part) and then expect to feel better, is an equation that doesn´t add up. The body gains from what we eat and what we do, but our thoughts also affect the body to a very high degree. Filling the body with negative or hateful thoughts is a self-harming behaviour, and we understand this when we learn more about how extremely great of an impact the thoughts have on the body.

To think of the body with love can be difficult to apply if we have migraines every day and feel desperate and ready to resort to any methods to get relief. But it´s not impossible to change a habitual thought pattern. As with much else, we have to decide, take the first step and stick to our intention. The more positive thoughts we have, the more we'll gain, as what we focus on grows stronger. It doesn´t matter if we think that we don´t want migraines or if we suppress our pain. We can´t focus anything away, we can only include what we want more of in our lives.

The next step to feeling better is to listen to the body's signals. As the body strives for balance, it will make you aware when things are not as they should be. Negative feelings and pain are the body's way of getting our attention, to get us to listen. I am convinced that most of us who have chronic migraines didn´t just get it from one day to another. The body has for a long time signaled that something is not okay, we´ve had more and more migraines, nausea, anxiety or maybe other symptoms, but we have often not taken the signals seriously and instead dismissed them. Since the body's task is to strive for balance, it has to do a bit more to reach us. Migraines effectively put us on hold. It literally holds us down. Unfortunately, this doesn´t always make us listen anyway. We try different medicines and treatments and sometimes we find the right one, the medicine works, and we feel happy and content. Unfortunately, this also often means that we just push the problem ahead, for example when we take medicine and go to work instead of resting. When the medicine then no longer works, the body continues to signal that something is wrong, but the symptoms are temporarily alleviated by medicine, so we are back to square one or even in a much worse condition because we have gone beyond our limits for what our body can handle. That is when we have "tried everything" and become desperate and depressed.

Listening to the body is not always easy when we have done everything we can for a long time to ignore it. Many of us have also learnt that if we don´t feel well, we should go to the doctor and he/she will make it better. Healthcare is fantastic in many ways and listening to the body doesn´t mean that we shouldn´t seek help if we need it. Nor does it mean that we shouldn´t take medicine if we need it. However, we need to take responsibility for our own part in the treatment. As a sufferer of migraines, it´s not uncommon for us to be exposed to different types of medication, and both doctors and nurses may well claim that we should continue to take a medication that doesn´t work and gives unpleasant side effects. Sometimes, of course, it can be during an escalation period, but it´s still important that we really make an active decision about this. In my repeated experience, not all doctors and nurses appreciate that patients listen to their body and have their own opinion, which surely many can relate to. In these situations, it´s important to be strong and stay focused. If this is difficult with a throbbing head, we can bring a person we trust as support when we have to convey our messages and opinions. When our entire body knows what´s right and wrong, we have to *follow that knowledge*. We should never be persuaded to go against our internal feelings, what we know deep down is right. In this context it´s also important to remember that since migraines affect millions of people, there is a market for all kinds of medicines and treatments as well as alternative methods that promise the world, but which are completely ineffective. If we become desperate enough, we can end up both paying for and listening to advice that leads us to overlook the body's signals, and the end result may well be that the head continues to ache in undiminished strength, the hopelessness is even greater, and the money has gone.

If we decide to really listen to the body, it can take time before we actually hear something. We are not used to it and don´t really know how it´s done, in addition, our mind might tell us that there is no point and a lot of other things that makes us doubt that it´s a feasible road.

What´s so amazing is that the body always gives us signals. The body doesn´t stop signalling to us just because we haven´t listened for 20 years, but we can start listening today. Now. Think of your body as your best friend who has the knowledge of your needs to feel better. The body knows what you need. Listen to the body as you listen to the one you love, with focus and attention.

To listen to the body also means that we may hear things we don´t want to hear, it may be that we need to make some change that affects others in the long run or something else that requires courage and determination. It´s in these situations that we must not forget that if we choose not to listen, life will not change, it will instead continue as usual. All change has consequences, and it means active decisions and choices.

If we don´t listen to the signals, it often ends with sick leave. Being on sick leave and resting does not usually mean that we thereafter can return to work full of energy and with the situation under control, but recovery in a conscious way is required on several levels. To live (not merely surviving) with migraines requires being aware of how to replenish energy, how we retain it and where we put its focus, so that our energy is always on the plus side. We need energy to change our lives. We need to calm our mind and put our thoughts on hold in order to let the good energy in.

So, how do you listen to the body? The first requirement is that our thoughts are still enough in order for us to hear. Sensations, feelings and pain are the body's way of communicating with us, but we have to be present enough in the moment to understand what it´s all about. We often feel like there are things we "have to" do; participate in various activities or just general life, but once we begin to perceive the body's signals, we might understand that our body needs to rest and therefore has other plans. This is when we need to be aware that we have a choice in what to prioritise. The body tells us what it is we need *right now*, not what we need later, in just a moment or another day. If we choose to listen, we slowly begin to recover and replenish energy. If we choose to rest *later*, it means that we push the recovery ahead of us, and the result is that it will probably take longer because the activity will take energy away from us, energy that we need for something else or energy that we really don´t have. Migraine is a disease that steals a lot of our time. Therefore, it can be difficult to rest when, for once, we may feel a little better. When we have a headache-free day, we want to take the opportunity to do everything we possibly can. A headache-free day is like winning the lottery. We also know that this price has a cost, many times it brings us straight back to the dark. The benefit of listening to the body and also resting on good days is that we produce strength to use when feeling worse, which in the end means that we recover faster.

If we listen to the body it won´t let us down, it is my experience and my absolute belief. We betray ourselves by not trusting that our body has an outstanding healing ability. The problem is that many of us lack the patience and knowledge to let the body heal at its own pace. We become desperate for relief and take medication or something else that is ultimately not good for us. It´s not our fault that we have migraines, but we are responsible for taking care of ourselves based on our circumstances. We only have one life and it's happening right now. We can´t expect to feel good if we ignore the body's signals. We can´t expect to recover in a just few weeks if we haven´t listened to the body's signals for several years. For most people with chronic migraines, there is no quick fix. Thankfully, there are good medicines that can help us go through the recovery, but as long as we put all our trust in medicine, we'll be dependent on it working. It´s not uncommon for the effect to diminish over time. If we have the patience to listen to the body, get to know the signals and to trust it, we will have our own control and knowledge of what we need, and not only be dependent on healthcare and / or other people or circumstances, but instead trust our own judgment of what we need. While we wait for the miracle medicine or something else that will make the migraine disappear, life goes on. Every day is valuable and will never come back. The most important thing of all is to find an approach and tools that allow us to participate in life here and now, regardless of whether we have migraines or not. I am living proof that this works.

Yoga and meditation took me on a journey that made me start listening to my body and heart. I knew nothing about yoga, it was blurry and strange to me, but at least it couldn´t get any worse. When I started yoga, everything gave me migraines. It wasn´t worthwhile to keep track of triggers, it was easier to keep track of what I didn´t get migraines from, for example, breathing or drinking a glass of water. My yoga debut started with a workout called "The Little Back Session", and I couldn´t even turn my body before I got cramps, I couldn´t bend my head before I got a migraine. I often laid down to just breathe and I called that yoga, it was the only thing I could do. I many times literally crawled to the yoga mat. It was claimed that 40 days was required to feel the effect, and that was my goal. I slowly began to hear what my body was telling me. It didn´t take long, but the most difficult thing was to *pursue* that message, because the power of habit is great and breaking thought patterns takes time. But I had no choice, I had no life.

Since I started listening to my body, amazing things have happened. Without any major effort, things I don´t feel good about have been phased out and things I need have been added, for example, when it comes to food and exercise. Yoga, meditation and breathing exercises have taught me to listen to my body, and it has given results beyond expectation. When I ran the 5 kilometres Spring Race without stopping, it was a victory bigger than many can understand. From feeling like a powerless, exhausted, depressed zombie with a knife in my head, I ran 5 kilometres. Since that day, I feel an even greater admiration for what my amazing body can accomplish. If we listen, changes naturally happen without struggle, judgement or a bad conscience. I am stronger today than I have been in 20 years!

It´s important to point out that listening to the body is not the same as being passive. Listening to the body is not really difficult at all, the biggest challenge and difficulty is to get the mind / thoughts to agree instead of putting sticks in the wheel.

TO ENJOY LIFE

Many of us with chronic migraines and a lot of pain have experience from mental illness. Many have been or are depressed and exhausted. It becomes a vicious circle - the pain triggers depression and depression trigger more pain. At the same time, there are many who witness that when they, for example, changed jobs or ended a relationship, their migraines got much better or even disappeared. Being at a job we don´t like, continuing with a relationship that deep inside doesn´t feel good, or constantly find ourselves in a place we deep down don´t like, creates internal stress, which in turn contributes to tension in the body. We can´t deal with these tensions by taking stress-relieving medications, going for a massage, resting or going on holiday. These measures may remove the symptoms for a while, but the basic problem remains. Nor is it always the case that we make the connection to our health. We deny that we don´t thrive or feel free and happy in certain situations and relationships, because it would mean big changes that we may not be able to cope with or that frighten us. Big changes often involve other people, people we love and care about. We don´t even want to think about the idea of disappointing others and instead choose to stay. We suppress our longing, and the body continues to protest. Eventually, the body becomes like a pressure cooker and the migraine thrives amongst the tension and denial.

There are probably many of us who have been told during a visit to the doctors that we are depressed, that we feel mentally unwell etc. It can often feel provoking because we believe that it´s the migraine and the pain that are causing our mental illness, and that can certainly be true, but I think it can be good to sometimes still think about whether it´s only the migraines that we can´t handle, or if in fact there may be other grounds as well. If we are to change a situation we don´t thrive in, we need to be honest with ourselves and have the courage to listen to what we deep down want and don´t want.

Most people who, despite all internal resistance, change their lives and break up from a negative situation and feel better, can in retrospect, with perspective, see that there have been times when they realised that the current situation is not what they really wanted. The insight has come at regular intervals but has been effectively pushed away and denied. Personally, I have met many people who state that they get migraines when they are not happy, and that the changes they have made have been necessary in order to feel better.

LET YOUR HEART LEAD THE WAY

Love and humour are the hearts way, and really the only way we need to go. I have always strived for simplicity and clarity to understand and to be able to stick to important lessons. I have found a way to easily describe how I have learnt to relate to the environment, to everything that might possibly show up on a daily basis. I have learnt this approach through yoga and meditation, and it helps me to stay calm, to focus, to let go of things, to be kinder to myself and to rejoice and enjoy life. Migraines are taking up less and less space in my life.

For us to feel good, I believe we have to start with what contributes to love, joy, energy, vitality, creativity and curiosity about life. Unconditional love lives in the heart, which means love free from prejudice, judgement, comparisons and criticism. When I use the word love, I mean love in a broader concept, love for our loved ones, but also love for our fellow human beings. Love for our fellow human beings can be to show compassion and support, to listen and be present, a pat on the shoulder when you are sad, etc.

Unconditional love that comes from the heart means a love that´s free from the fact that circumstances must be a certain way for us to feel it. A good example of this is by looking at an important loved one who´s unconditionally loved simply because he/she exists. The heart knows when we act out of love for ourselves and respect for our own worth. When we act on the basis of self-love and respect for our own worth, we feel good and our entire body feels good, when we go *against* the heart, accuse ourselves, feel ashamed that we have migraines or whatever it may be, our bodies don´t feel particularly good and we don´t feel well. In this way, the heart leads the way to where we need to go to in order to feel increasingly better. The clever thing is that when we listen to the heart, all the good spreads to our surroundings. I will explain with a couple of examples:

Example 1:
You´re at work and things are going well now that you have a plan for how to cope with a whole working day and keeping the stress in check, and therefore also the migraine. It feels good, you find confidence in the future. One day when arriving to work a bit later, just like you had agreed with the boss, one of the colleagues comes up to you and tells you that you are in fact not the only one at work with a headache, there are several more, so why do you get a free pass?

How do you react to this?
Option 1: You get sad and feel misunderstood and run over, you may think this person is an idiot who should keep quiet, he/she does not understand that there is a difference between a migraine and headache, sigh. Or something like that. You start defending yourself and soon the day is ruined. You feel sad and maybe go to the toilet and cry in secret. You get back into the mind frame of a victim.

Option 2: You consult the heart. The heart that conveys unconditional love tells you that this person may not be well, this person may have had a sleepless night, you know that he/she has small children. The heart shows you that this is not about you, but about the other person's inner struggle. So instead of defending yourself, you say for example, that it was sad that he/she perceived the situation that way. You might say that if he/she has a lot of headaches, the boss is great at giving support, so the work situation should become good for him/her as well.

In option one, you begin to defend and excuse yourself, hence giving your power and dignity to the other. You think negative thoughts about the other, which means that you hurt yourself in the long run, because we now know what negative thoughts do to the body. You increase your inner stress.

In option two, you retain your power over the situation. You show compassion for another person who may need a break at work, which might lay a seed in the other person resulting in him/her changing their situation. You keep your mood at a steady level, you keep calm and the stress under control.

To ask the heart a question doesn´t mean that we should become weak and let people walk all over us, absolutely not. Asking the heart means that we should become aware of the times we put ourselves down and gave away our power and dignity. Asking the heart means that we follow the path to feeling better, because when we maintain our power and dignity, we act accordingly and evolve. When we give up our power and dignity, we become victims and end up staying where we are and instead continue to suffer.

Things happen when we start asking the heart for guidance, both in our body and surroundings. If we listen to the heart, we feel better, which benefits everyone around us. The family will become happy if we feel better, we´ll feel calmer because we learn not to get started on things that have nothing to do with us. In the long run, it also means that major changes can take place without anxiety, such as changing jobs or changing other situations we don´t like. Asking the heart for guidance is a process that never ends. Asking the heart is a lifelong learning experience, but it´s also a great way to evolve and experience life. My heart guided me to the Sahara where my life turned. It has guided me to Puerto Rico to dance and meet strong and amazing women who also listen to their hearts and who gave me lifelong friendships. My heart has guided me to meetings with wise people who have taught me a lot about life, and who in various ways have helped me let go of migraines and suffering. My heart has taught me to listen to my inner creativity, which enriches my life on so many levels, and which has meant that I can choose to work differently and avoid stress.

TO DISTINGUISH BETWEEN EMOTIONS AND PAIN

My whole life turned when I realised that I could distinguish between my emotions and my pain. For a long time, I had been practicing yoga and meditation, I had been resting and listening to my body and feeling much better. I was starting to get more and more energy, but I still had a lot of migraines and tension headaches. One day I realised I was happy! I was happy for no reason, just like that. It was at that moment I realised that I was done letting the migraine control my life and that I had made a choice. I had decided to be happy regardless of the migraines.

From that day on, I began to focus more consciously on what I wanted more of in life and I finally let go of the migraines altogether, something I had talked about many times in CBT therapy, but it was only now that the token fell down. Letting go of the migraine doesn´t mean that I *suppressed* that I have one, to suppress something is not the same as letting go because constriction creates tension. I let go of the migraine by *giving up the fight* against it. I had been fighting the migraine for many years and it was pointless. I would never win. I gave up, it could be there if it wanted to. I realised I was missing out on life while struggling. I wanted to live, I wanted to be happy and enjoy my life.

Focusing on what you want more of in your life and having a positive attitude towards life, despite the headaches, requires training and patience. It takes confidence in life and to let go of the control of things having to be a special way in order to feel good. It requires living consciously by constantly making active choices, several times a day, taking responsibility for your own feelings and reactions and getting to know yourself. It requires living in the present. It also requires acceptance and self-love, not to judge, criticise or beat yourself up when, despite all the insights, you are suddenly back on square one and curse the whole world for the hell of migraines. Once we have experienced the power of focusing, we get back on our feet much faster because we know what works.

To me, there is no reasonable doubt that if we are to achieve what we want, what we want most of all, we must reverse the whole reasoning. Most people who suffer from chronic migraines think, as far as I know, that when the cure comes, you will engage in life, do the things you long to do. You will do it *later*, when times get better. And the days go by, that turn into months and soon into years. In the meantime, life goes by. By reversing the reasoning and focusing on a better feeling, on things you want in your life, you are not dependent on whether the cure comes tomorrow or in 10 years. If you create the feeling that what we want most of all has already happened, you can enjoy life regardless, despite pain. And the migraine and pain end up in the background because the struggle is over.

Distinguishing between emotions and pain is easier said than done if we don´t know how it´s done. Admittedly, it´s only us that control how we should feel, and we do so through our thoughts. Migraines and the pain that it causes often contribute to negative thoughts that contribute to feelings of fear, hopelessness and helplessness, or anger and bitterness, and then the negative spiral continues, and we aggravate our pain, the physical, but also our inner pain. It´s not the migraine itself that is the cause of the negative thoughts and feelings, but our thoughts are often the result of years of the same repeated thoughts, and the power that´s in these negative thoughts takes time to break.

There are many ways to break negative thoughts and other destructive patterns that cause us harm. From my experience, it can be difficult, even provocative, when someone claims that you can be happy even though your head hurts. Anyone who says that probably doesn´t know how awful it is to have a migraine or is stuck in some kind of denial stage. But I claim, with my own experience with the migraines from hell and having tried to cure them with denial, that it works. It actually works beyond all expectations. This is where we need to start really getting our lives and zest for life back. Take back power over our lives.

When something feels difficult, it can be helpful to find another way to approach the subject, a way that is not loaded with questioning and negative perceptions. Believe that your feelings are energy!

EMOTIONS AND ENERGY

If we think that emotions and energy are the same thing, we can get around the problem of what´s possible and not possible to control. When emotions and energy are the same, it´s not difficult to understand that when we are happy, we are full of energy and we feel light and absorb our surroundings in a positive way. When we are depressed and sad, we feel powerless, our mind feels heavy and maybe even our body. We have no energy. We may prefer to be alone and we can´t cope with people who don´t understand how difficult things are for us.

With simple tricks we can raise our energy and thereafter our emotional state, and when practicing this several times a day it will become gradually easier.

There are two things involved here, one is that we train ourselves in a positive approach in the long term, at the same time as we adapt a "quick fix" in the moment. Just like with the negative thoughts that have been built up over a long period of time and become powerful because we´ve had our focus on them, we are now starting to focus on increasing the energy (to focus more on positive feelings), in a way where we partly have our own power to influence our feelings and being, and partly that joy should have more place in our lives. As these thoughts become more powerful, the negative thoughts increasingly lose their power. The idea of learning to raise our energy, hence our emotional state, is to first become aware of the negative thoughts at the moment and then immediately break them. To be able to do this, we need different tools.

In order for us to raise our energy and positive emotions, *all* means are allowed, i.e., all means subjecting that we are able to look at ourselves in the mirror afterwards and feel proud of how fantastic we are to bring out the power and do good things for ourselves. We can examine which means suit us individually. An easy way to raise energy immediately involves breathing exercises and to move the body. We can do some yoga exercises, dance for a while, stretch, walk, swim, walk in the woods, play, laugh, pet the cat or anything that feels good and that we are able to do. When we move the body, serotonin is stimulated, which contributes to us feeling better. Having a strategy that helps us raise energy, hence the possibility of feeling better, is extremely helpful and this strategy doesn´t have to be complicated or difficult.

As with all changes, it´s important to start from where we currently stand. It´s unlikely that going from feeling depressed, tired and sad, we'll suddenly start feeling a zest for life, joy and happiness, and to soon thereafter wanting all the challenges in the world. However, we need a direction forward, even if that means we have to start by deep breathing on the yoga mat because that's the only thing that works. We simply have to get energy and lift our spirits to be able to feel better in the long run.

Just as there are energy-boosting activities, there are opposites. Things that take our energy away and that ultimately leads to a mood drop, things that make us depressed and feel worse. These are things we do out of old habit or that we think lead to more energy. Again, this is another good time to gauge how we feel on the inside, but also to consider whether it´s something we risk regretting afterwards. I´m thinking of eating sweets or something else that contributes to a temporary increase in energy, but which in the long run worsen our mood. How many times have we not eaten something to numb our emotions and in hindsight feel guilty? This also applies to activities such as gossiping, blaming others, judging and generally speaking negatively about ourselves and others. Sure, in the moment it might feel good talking about it, but it's treacherous. It´s unlikely that we can look at ourselves in the mirror with pride over the fact that we have gossiped about others or blamed ourselves. Gossip and negative talk create an inner stress. It´s extremely important that we stay out of whining and complaints, both our own and others'. It´s a safe way to prevent us from running out of energy and becoming exhausted.

We need to be uncompromising with our energy. Migraine itself takes a lot of energy and we have to make do with what we have, be sure that we take more energy in than we give out. We do this by becoming aware of how we bring energy home and where and to whom we give it. We also need to make sure we replenish energy every day in whatever way possible. We many times wait until the weekend, or for when we´re free, and that doesn´t work because we continuously need new energy to keep our body balanced. Our body doesn´t care when there is a free space in the diary, our body is here. Right now.

THE POWER OF THOUGHTS

When people around us say that we have to think positive and other similar things to this, it´s easy to feel that this person doesn´t understand anything. Unfortunately, positive thinking has become worn out and is used without a thought for anything else. If we let go of the preconceptions against this statement for a while, and think about what it means to think positively, we discover the power in it. When the positive thinking goes deep and becomes a positive attitude, a healthy optimism mixed with self-love and humour, miracles can happen. Then it's powerful! If we train ourselves to focus on positive thinking and attitudes, we are halfway to the goal. Note that this doesn´t mean that we should repress or deny our situation or the reality we live in, that´s when positive thinking becomes the shallow clichés that we can´t stand.

So, what is positive thinking that goes deeper and becomes a positive approach? My experience and interpretation are that it´s a thought process that needs to be trained until it becomes the obvious in life, but one that also needs to be maintained. We can always fall back into negative thoughts if we don´t look out. Therefore, we need to practice taking care of ourselves, and make reasonable demands on what we can handle. We don´t have to take everything so seriously, life can be very comical in the midst of all the misery.

Becoming aware of one's attitude requires that we get to know ourselves and our reactions, and that we find the voice of our heart, i.e., the love and care for ourselves. It´s only when we listen to our heart, instead of the old negative thoughts that easily can appear when we´ve done something "wrong", that we can choose. As an example, I have an endless number of times forgotten important things and kicked myself for it, considered myself a bad mother, a bad colleague and all sorts of things. I have become angry and disappointed in myself, which in the end resulted in migraines and suffering. When I´ve become aware that I can actually choose a different approach, meaning that I see myself as a competent and valuable person that do the best I can, the result is completely different. Even though I still have forgotten what I was supposed to remember, I avoid headaches and feeling guilty, because I know that I have done everything I could, based on current circumstances. This also means that I can let go of mistakes I have made. It´s when we feel that we could´ve done differently or that we hurt someone else that the feelings of guilt thrive, and we dwell on the same thing to try to justify something that has already happened.

A positive attitude is extremely important, even in difficult situations that are not only about dealing with stress and chaos in everyday life, but when we train our thoughts and our attitude, we can also handle situations that are about deep fears, severe pain, anxiety and uncertainty. When we start to become aware of how much difference it actually makes how we relate to different situations, not just intellectually, we discover how much we can influence how we feel. Life is full of situations we can´t control, but we can choose how to relate to them. The most important thing is that we make that choice *before* the situation arises. Once we are there, it´s much harder to choose.

THE UNDERSTANDING FROM PEOPLE AROUND US

It´s important to spread knowledge about migraines so that everyone affected has the same opportunities for specialist care, work and rehabilitation. When it comes to the understanding from people around us on a more personal, individual level, such as family, friends and work colleagues, I think like this; first of all, a person that´s never had an attack can´t understand what it´s like to have a migraine, so we can´t expect them to actually understand the pain, the feeling or the anxiety. In addition, migraines are not visible, so when we´re amongst people we usually look quite okay, which makes it even more difficult for non-sufferers to understand how bad it can actually be. This is not really strange because if we look at another example, people with two healthy legs can´t understand what it can be like to live paralysed from the waist down. We can show consideration, we can have compassion and try to support as best we can, but we can never fully understand another person's experience or what it´s like to live with one or the other condition.

In our society, there are many diseases, diagnoses, disabilities and conditions that require understanding and compassion. Just like we who are affected by migraines need to spread knowledge, the same applies to, for example, people with diabetes, people with mental illness or people with other diseases and conditions. There are several associations and subjects that require understanding, it´s not the knowledge itself that is the problem, there is an endless amount of knowledge available on everything we need to know. The understanding we seek is the understanding and consideration that *everyone* seeks, which deviates from the so-called normal, or actually, from all people really. An understanding that is about avoiding prejudices and condemnations for things people don´t understand, which may evoke fear. To avoid people's opinions about things they have nothing to do with. That we are okay however we are. My view is that if we are to create an understanding of migraines, we need to stand up straight and stop being ashamed. There is nothing to be ashamed of, we have not gotten a migraine to avoid working or taking care of our children. We have suffered from migraines the same way others suffer from other things. But if we *act* like victims, apologise for our illness, work even though we should rest, or ignore the signals from the body and heart because we´re afraid what others will think, or because others don´t understand, then the result we don´t want is the result we´ll get, we leave our power and our dignity to people and circumstances around us. As long as we wait for someone else to change their behaviour to make us feel better, we make ourselves victims. We can´t control other people (luckily), but we can decide how to relate to our surroundings. There will always be people who don´t take us into account, but they should not be allowed to control or limit our lives.

I think many people are good at informing their colleagues about what it means to have a migraine, the suffering it gives and how much energy it takes. But what happens if, after all the information, we still go to work even though we are not in a condition to work at all, even though we have by far crossed the line and stay upright only due to painkillers and all the other tricks we usually use? What do we teach our colleagues? We teach them that it´s probably not as bad as we claim. We teach them that we may be exaggerating a little when we explain how terrible the pain can be, how we lie in bed and vomit in a dark room and then still show up to work. We ask the impossible of our colleagues if we say one thing and do another. How should those who have never had a migraine understand? It's not possible. What we send out is what we get back, it´s a simple basic universal law. If we want to change the view of people affected by migraines, of ourselves, we have to start with us!

Let´s think of a workplace. We have a job that we enjoy, but sometimes the impressions become too much, we get tired, stressed and when we get home all our energy is gone and we can´t do anything else for the rest of the day because our head hurts. The next morning, we might have a migraine when we wake up, we end up taking medicine and then head to work. The days continue like this until the day we have to call in sick, we can´t postpone the migraine anymore. We may stay at home for 1-2 days before returning to work. Then we start from square one again. Does anyone recognise themself? On all the occasions we have to call work and report sick we get a bad feeling in our stomach, bad conscience, feelings of guilt, maybe a little anxiety about staying at home once again, that colleagues get a bigger workload due to our absent.

Let´s look at it from another point of view. We figure out what´s needed from us to have the energy to work a whole day without it resulting in migraines and time spent in dark rooms during our spare time on weekends and holidays. In this way, we take power over the situation, we take responsibility for listening to the body and we are able to work. We inform the workplace what migraines are about and how it affects us. We tell them what we need to be able to do the job and agree with the boss on how this should best work. There are probably many who have already done this, but the point is that you then just have to stick to the plan without explaining, defending or apologising! We stick to the plan without judging or having a bad conscience because we do what we have to. If we begin to *explain, defend or apologise* for sticking to the plan we have decided on, we become victims. We have already explained. The boss knows. End of. We have to show that our worth does not come from how much we adapt to what others think and feel, but that we are all different, and that it´s okay. We don´t appreciate our own worth if we start apologising for wanting to look after ourselves so that we can work and have a good life. On the contrary, an illness like migraine, which really requires us to listen to the body, can help us learn other important things about life. Because by sticking to the plan, we can teach our colleagues how important it is to take care of yourself when you have a migraine. We can teach them that it's okay to take a break when it's stressful. We can teach them that our needs are important. By respecting our needs, we teach our fellow human beings that when *they* feel unwell for some reason, it's okay for *them* to take responsibility and to take care of themselves. Most people are kind and wish others well, and by showing that we actually want to be their colleagues, that we take our responsibility to make sure we´re able to work together and do our part of the job, we get consideration and respect back. The plan applies even if there now happens to be a colleague that starts whining about us potentially getting an extra day off when he/she still has to work. We need to just let it run off us like water off a duck's back, and then stand up straight because this can be a critical point for us where we could potentially come off track. It´s suitable to have a good strategy here (which we have decided on in advance) to encourage ourselves.

If, after all, there are days when we still have to call in sick, it evokes a completely different feeling. The boss and colleagues have a knowledge of migraines and know what is required of us. They know there is a plan. They know we're following the plan. Then they also know that when we call in sick, it´s serious. Then we don´t have to lie at home with a bad conscience because we "disappoint" our colleagues, we know they are aware we have taken care of ourselves. The rest is not at our disposal. When we take responsibility, we release a lot of our anxiety and fear. When we take responsibility, we regain our strength and our dignity. When we take responsibility, we are not victims.

If we try to make others understand how much we suffer by presenting ourselves as victims of a terrible illness, there is a great risk we´ll be perceived as whiny or that we exaggerate. Because a person who doesn´t have migraines can´t possibly know how terrible the pain can be, they can believe anything. Most people who have an illness or a problem and behave like victims, believe they are suffering the most. We think that having a migraine is one of the biggest sufferings you can have. Others think, for example, that having a stomach ulcer or a man who is unfaithful is the worst suffering you can have. Everyone thinks that the difficulties they go through are the worst suffering you can have. *You can´t compare ways of suffering!* Our worth does not lie in how much or how little we suffer. We are all worth equally in whatever disease or circumstance we live with.

Furthermore, I think it´s the same starting point that applies in private life. We inform and talk to our loved ones, give them knowledge and describe things as much as we can for them to understand, but I think it´s also important to set a limit here. When important and beloved people around us have the knowledge of migraines and we have told them what it means for us, we then shouldn´t have to continue to explain ourselves, defend and apologise. I believe that it´s devastating for our well-being to put migraines in focus all the time. It doesn´t have to be in focus, we won´t forget that we have migraines. It´s what we want more of in our lives that needs to be in focus. In any case, my point is that there is a big difference between saying that you need to go and rest for a while, to just actually do it (because we know that the others are aware of why), or to start explaining, defending and apologising for the fact that you have to rest and to remind them of migraines. Does it matter, you might be wondering then. Undoubtedly yes, if you ask me. To explain, defend and excuse ourselves because we need to take care of ourselves sends us straight back to the negative thoughts, suffering and ultimately the victim position. We don´t have to explain, defend or apologise to *anyone* that we have a migraine and that we need to take care of ourselves because in practice this means that we ask permission from people around us to do what makes us feel good. And we don´t need anyone else's permission. Asking for permission means that we give someone else the power to approve and, in this way, we diminish ourselves and give away our power and dignity. We need no one's approval for anything, however, we often need to be kinder to ourselves. I want to emphasise that I don´t mean that we should hide having migraines, absolutely not. It´s important to spread knowledge and information, but it´s also important to think about the purpose of highlighting migraines as a cause of certain behaviours. Is the purpose to inform or to get an approval?

Finally, I would like to emphasise that, of course, it´s not easy to change attitudes, it takes time and patience. If we come to the conclusion that we want to change our attitude, we need to surround ourselves with people who support and encourage, and who can provide constructive feedback, so that we don´t stand alone against all the unpleasant challenges. Changing one's attitude is challenging and requires courage and determination, but the gain is a wonderful feeling of freedom and victory that leads to energy and better health. Meeting others who suffer from migraines to support each other and feel connected can be very rewarding and enjoyable. However, my most important experience and biggest warning flag is that sometimes these groups can lead us to not move an inch towards our desire to feel better, because when the conversations of comparing suffering and injustice stop, we are undoubtedly stuck in the victim position and there is no energy or power left for changes. I have experienced it many times and it leads to nowhere further than to the confirmation of our suffering. But if you, with the support of the group behind you, have the courage to challenge yourself and make room to grow and evolve, it can be worth its weight in gold. It's like having a big safe hug to come back to and rest in after exploring on unknown territories for some time. People cheer you on and love comes your way, and confirmation of there being hope for a better quality of life and that you can actually influence your life. And success breeds success, by self-development, but also being present when others develop themselves is very rewarding and instructive. Taking back power over life is the only way to feeling better.

MOVE YOUR BODY - THE POWER OF HABIT

We all know by now how important it is to move the body and how difficult it can be for us to find the motivation and get started. During the worst attacks, of course, it´s not possible, but as soon as we can stand up, we can move.

Finding the motivation doesn´t mean that we can just sit or lie on the couch and wait for it to fall down on us. However, we can kill the motivation by trying too hard so that we instead feel bad, get a bad attack and just hate everything that exercise and workouts are called. It becomes increasingly harder to get to grips with things, we find explanations, we are either too unwell to move, our migraine is too severe, or we get dizzy etc. Breaking habitual patterns is difficult for everyone. There is a security and a predictability in the way things are, even if it´s pain and fatigue, depression and a bad conscience. The positive thing is that we have the power to change our lives in many different ways ourselves, and if the life we live on a day to day is not the life we want, we have to start changing ourselves. No one can change our lives for us.

The first thing we have to do is to realise our starting point with self-love. We were perhaps sporty in the past, were fit and could run, cycle and climb trees. Today, we have run out of energy or decreased drastically, but we hold on to the past and plan our workouts according to an unrealistic picture that evokes demands for performance and results. Therefore, it´s important to let go of the old image and focus on here and now. Honestly and clearly, lovingly and without paraphrasing, we ask ourselves what we can do right now. Start small, almost too small, it quickly becomes a success and when we make progress, we are encouraged to continue a little longer.

As a goal, start by moving on certain days of the week, let's say five days a week. Make a success diary where everything that is more than nothing is a success. Everything counts and anything beyond the five days is a bonus! Find the way you feel you can move, it doesn´t matter what it is, just that it happens. It can be anything from walking three laps around the house, walking the children to school, cycling to the local supermarket, going for a powerwalk, swimming or riding or anything that means you move a little more than usual. A very simple trick can be to use a step-counter. Determine the number of steps you should take per day five times a week. If you walk more steps than you have decided on, or if you do anything else in addition to this, it´s a bonus, if you cycle or dance for example. This should also be included in the success diary. All means are allowed for you to be encouraged by the diary and continue. Use crayons, happy stickers and more. Make a summary once a week and when you feel that it´s quite easy to reach your goal, you increase it a little more. Remember that this is not a competition. Remember not to put yourself down if you end up on the couch again despite all the good intentions. Observe your thoughts and what triggered the negative spiral, think of it as an experience and thank yourself for learning something new about yourself. Get up and continue the next day. It´s important that we pay attention to the success and remind ourselves why we do this and why we have patience. If we´ve had migraines and been exhausted for a long period of time, it will take a while before things turns around and feel like something we want to do voluntarily. Since this is about changing a (bad) habit and doing something else, both your body and your mind will struggle, sometimes very hard. As long as we move in a conscious, empathetic and realistic way, just keep going. Try not to focus on whether the migraine is getting better or worse, focus on what you want, on the positive effects that will arise.

Anyone who tells themself that the migraine gets better from being still has only fallen into the trap created by the ego to stay in the same familiar state. Migraines will never get better from being still. At the same time, it´s a balancing act, on one hand to recover strength by resting and sleeping enough, and on the other hand by moving the body to become stronger. The point is to find a way to move the body that feels good, that feels strengthening and that in fact in the long run can very well mean that we long for movement and based on that feel how the body becomes stronger and more flexible.

I have gone from being totally exhausted with the migraine from hell to longing to run, dance, do yoga and many other things. I have energy and my body feels strong, and I now appreciate my body just as it is. Of course, I have headaches and migraines sometimes, a little pain here and there, but it belongs to everyday life and nowadays it's about not listening properly. It's usually about stress and negative thoughts, but it passes when I listen and focus on my needs.

It has taken several years to get to where I am today. Once I decided to change my life, I tried over and over again to get started with some kind of exercise, but many times ended up in the achievement trap and everything became a big mess. In the end, I let go of the demands, got tired of pushing myself and instead decided on three things; Yoga and meditation every day, if only for 5 minutes, walking at least 30 minutes a day (because I have a dog it was a must), writing in my success diary and throwing the migraine diary away. I sometimes walked and moved a little extra, wrote in the success diary, smothered myself in my successes, encouraged myself, cheered myself on and thought about how strong I was. The walks continued to get longer and one day (after about 2 years) I suddenly wanted to run! I felt like running, I still feel like running. And dance. And swim. And ride. I never force myself to exercise anymore, I want to! I feel good about it. It makes me happy. I'm getting strong. I stand up straight. It´s rare that I get a migraine before or after exercise, but if I get one, I take care of myself without putting any thought to it. I know what I need. After exercising, it´s wonderful to rest, lie on the couch and read and just enjoy.

Together we are strong. When we find other people who share the same desire and the wish to feel better and have more energy, we can get fantastic support to help break habits on the way. If we support each other's successes together and show love and support for each other, we can more easily get out of the weaknesses we sooner or later get stuck in. A support group where we can be just the way we are, where everything is okay and we evolve at our own pace. In addition to the fact that we can sometimes get a (loving) kick in the butt, we also learn from each other what it means not having to achieve something in any way or to fix something, we are worthy just as we are. It gives a ripple effect on our everyday life. The crucial thing is that we gently but firmly help each other to move away from having the mind frame of a victim and remind each other that we have the power to change our lives. Another great way to spur yourself on is to speak to others. Many of us are good at talking about our limitations (stop that!), but now is the time to reverse the trend. When we speak to people around us and tell them that we ´ve started exercising, we get positive feedback from those who want to see us develop and anyone with doubts gets phased out. The reason why it´s good to speak to people is because we then concentrate on our focus and feelings. We feel a bit proud and that means more than we sometimes understand. We change direction on our future, even if we only manage to walk around the house twice a week. Suddenly, the desire will run an extra lap and then we´ll smother ourselves in happiness and success! It´s important that we find something that feels fun to do, even if it´s not the ideal according to common perceptions. The most important thing is to get started. Be curious and try something new.

WHAT DO YOU NEED TO HEAL?

If we are to be healed in the long run, we need to ask ourselves the question what we are prepared to change in order to be healed. How much do we want it? Do we have the courage? If you had to move to feel good, would you do it? Could you imagine ending certain relationships to feel good? Would you change jobs? Changing one's life requires determination and courage, but also confidence in life. When we change and make new choices, we turn and go a new way towards the unknown. Brave and with a straight back, we have to embrace the unknown and trust ourselves, turn to our inner strength and move forward. We must focus on the way forward, the feeling of already feeling better and letting go of the fear and the familiar, what we leave behind. If we really want a different life, a different future, it´s one foot in front of the other. The ego and mind will struggle, probably also the people around you. A good way is to practice doing things we don´t really have the courage to do, small things that on the whole may not seem so significant, but which contribute to greater confidence in ourselves.

The body doesn´t know the difference between saying no to someone or to go parachuting, it gives the same worrying feeling in the stomach and the same palpitations, sweating and other symptoms. If we thereby practice challenging ourselves little at a time, moving the boundaries of our comfort zone, we'll suddenly realise that we have taken several steps forward onto our new unknown path. Every time we do something we don´t actually have the courage to do, we grow stronger, we embrace our own power, we honour our value, we create a new future, we break patterns, we encourage ourselves, we grow as people, we evolve, we become stronger, we increase our self-awareness and our experience by having power over our lives.

It is not always easy to do things we don´t have the courage to do, for example, if we say no to someone we used to say yes to and the person in question reacts in a negative way, it can feel as if it wasn´t worth it. Or if we challenge ourselves and get migraines. Therefore, it´s important that even before we challenge ourselves, we prepare and repeat to ourselves why we do this. If our challenge of wanting to change and take responsibility for our own lives come from a genuine desire from the heart, any negative expressions from the environment will be about other people's fears of change. Remember that we are not responsible for other people's reactions. Our goal and our intention are not to feel better at someone else's expense.

Challenging oneself is not just about doing new things, it's mainly about turning inwards and to listen. Many of us who suffer from migraines are ambitious and active, which in many cases has been a contributing factor for us not stopping ourselves in time. A big challenge can be to do *nothing*, to just be, to sit and breathe and experience what´s happening. Challenging yourself by *not* performing, *not* being active, can be the most difficult, but also the absolute best. Activity and performance can often be an escape from something that hurts, something that we don´t want to feel, some old fear that we haven´t let go of, and that causes inner tension and pain. It can also be a dream, something we long for, but which we don´t allow ourselves to feel because we think we can´t get there.

Changing direction in life, moving towards something that is currently the unknown, means that we also have to let go of expectations of results and just be. That´s the key to healing.
This is also great to practice in a support group. It's easier to remind each other to persevere, to have trust, if we do it together. Healing needs space in our lives and it doesn´t fit if the space is occupied by expectations, impatience, control and performance anxiety.

Taking the step from a well-known everyday life and changing direction requires, as I said, focus, courage and trust. We many times get stuck in thoughts such as "if I do migraine yoga for 40 days *how* will it help me feel better?" We want guarantees, control over how things should help us, preferably in advance. The point of embracing the unknown is also about letting go of how things should work out exactly, how the body should heal and so on. Our focus must be on why we want to heal and then we have to focus on the feeling of feeling good, that is, being happy, have a clear head, having energy, feeling love and joy and everything else amazing that life consists of.

THE ENDING

I hope this book has given you hope that life can be amazing despite migraines and that you have the power to create the life you desire. Start where you are, one thing at a time and make the most of each day. Focus on what you want more of in your life and let go of control as much as you can. I wish you good luck with all my heart.

I end by sharing some diary notes.

Notes from 2011 - 2016

"The Knife"
Waking up early in the morning, it's still dark. The head aches. The knife cuts behind the eye. The pain is sharp and intense. I move and the knife cuts. I feel a pair of warm feet pressed against my thighs. Beloved child, when did you crawl into bed? I feel the warm little body next to mine. I feel an intense moment of the endless love for my child. Please, can I just lie here in the warmth and fall asleep again. Let me get rid of the knife. I have to get up. I stand slowly. Stumble and fumble. The sounds and movements send missiles of pain to the head. Water and tablets. I sit down at the kitchen table and light the candles. All I hear is the wind, the time ticking in seconds and the breathing of loved ones. How many times have I sat like this? I know what to expect. A new day lies ahead of me. What I make of it is what it will turn out to be. What I planned will not come true. The knife holds its grip. I choose to fill my day with silence, without demands and achievements. Just be. That's good enough, that's my life. I don´t know how long I sit at the kitchen table. The pain subsides. I crawl into bed again, close to my beloved, with my arms around, the warmth and calm from the child fills me with a peace of mind

and happiness.

"A vacation from hell"
We met with relatives, as we often do in the summers. We thrive together, it
´s usually cosy, we hang out, talk and plan some excursions. Laugh a lot,
walk and cook in large quantities. The children love their cousins and are out
all day long. But that summer was a nightmare. The migraine didn´t want to
let go. I barely wanted to go on holiday, I felt that I couldn´t cope with many
people, at the same time I wanted to go so badly. The family didn´t want to
go without me. I followed. It was a summer to remember and to forget at the
same time. To remember because it should never be repeated. Forget because
it was so terribly difficult, and I just felt so bad. I was lying in a dark room
with the migraine from hell wanting to die. I cried and cried every day. Tried
to get up and talk a little. There was pain, anxiety and nausea in a single
chaos. Had to go to bed again. Heard all the sounds from loved ones through
the thin wall, who hadn´t seen each other for a long time and they talked,
joked and laughed. The little girls who had longed for me, who think I am a
fantastic and funny aunt, they missed me even though I was there. The little
girls who wanted to bake a cake with me which we then would take
photographs of. I could not bear them. I was in so much pain, I was restless,
the anxiety had an iron grip around my lungs. In the end, I went out in sheer
desperation. I walked and walked and walked. Mile after mile, fast, quickly
away from it all, I wanted to feel so exhausted that I would fall asleep and get
away from everything. I was really not to anyone's delight. I didn´t know
what to do. I was in the prison of hell from pain and anxiety. The only thing I
knew was that I never wanted to feel so bad again. Either do everything to
have a better life or the alternative. Fall asleep. Avoid feeling. An option that
was not an option. But that was the only consolation, that the resort was
always there.

"The journey"
I had decided. I give myself another year, if I don´t feel better I will choose
the only way out. The resort that was the only consolation. I had no life. I
couldn´t take it anymore. I didn´t want to live in the hell of pain and anxiety
anymore. I had tried everything, countless medications. Like a guinea pig. I
heard about migraine yoga, I had never tried yoga. It could not make my life

worse, so I started. Or whatever you might call me doing. The Little Back-Session, the basic workout of migraine yoga. It went so-so. I got migraines when I bowed my head, cramps when I twisted my body and I hated Breath of fire. But I did it. Every day for 40 days. Or not really. Some days I couldn´t get out of bed. I crawled to the yoga mat. Breathing. I called it yoga. Slowly I got a little bit better. Yoga helped, not the pain, but the mind. I got a few seconds of peace of mind. So, I continued a little longer. And got a little more peace of mind. I started singing the mantra, the chaos in my head was put on hold. Good. I continued. Some days I wanted to give up, but there was no alternative. Just darkness. I started a course. And one more. One day I received a letter in the post. A card with some people sitting in the desert meditating. In close contact with Mother Earth. A yoga trip to the Sahara. My heart said yes.

Go! I wanted to so badly. But how would I cope with chronic migraine? Some days I couldn´t get up. I called and talked to one of the yoga teachers. You were supposed to gather in Marrakesh, the journey to the Sahara crossed the mountains in an off-road car and we would travel in the evening. Sit in the car all night on winding roads and be there in the morning. Rest one day. Hike in the desert and live in tents. Primitive. Without running water, just bring the essentials. It sounded great and challenging, but it wouldn´t work. I would not be able to. I would get sick, get a migraine, vomit on the way, get anxiety and miss home. But I wanted to. I felt that this would help me find myself under all layers of illness, pain and hopelessness. I asked myself what the worst thing that could happen was.

That I got a migraine and everything that comes with it. I realised that it didn´t matter because I would get it regardless. I got a migraine from everything. If I wanted to follow my heart, I couldn´t let the migraine limit me. I was facing a decision. I was terribly scared. The thoughts of disaster took turns. And what would everyone else think? All other healthy people who would join. What if I became a burden? I will never forget what the yoga teacher said. Words that finally sank into my heart. "Maria, everything is ok just as it is. We deal with what happens. Only you can decide if you should go along". I looked in the mirror. Have I not always seen myself as a brave person? Without fret, I embark on anything and everyone. I'm not scared. But this was different. It was not just a trip to the Sahara, it was a trip to my inner self. Over mountains and through fears. Embrace Mother Earth and let me be held, give up trying to have everything a certain way. I could choose. Dare, or stay in what I didn´t want to be in. I closed my eyes, took a deep breath and said yes. I went. It was amazing. I was forced to give up all my attempts to control the circumstances. My life turned. From that day on, life got better. And by day, it continues to get better. Because I found courage and started shifting my focus to opportunities instead of limitations.

"Freedom"
The automatic door slowly closed behind me. I took a few steps to the side, closed my eyes and stretched my arms towards the blue spring sky. Filled the lungs with the crisp spring air. The sun's gentle lukewarm rays dried the remnants of my tears. One more breath. It was as if the healthy clear breath spread throughout the body, from the feet, up to the stomach, the heart and finally the head. I lowered my arms. Opened my eyes in surprise and felt an intense presence. Suddenly everything was clear to me. I had just left the neurologist at the University Hospital and had seen a migraine specialist. I stood amongst the crowd of people walking in and out of the glass doors of the giant building that contains so much knowledge, experience and helping hands. Every now and then the realisation came that this was the last time. The last time anyone would tell me what my life was like. That would demand things of me that I didn´t want. That would tell me who I am. Take this medicine. Do this. Don´t do that. Do as the specialist say otherwise you will continue to have migraines and a poor quality of life. I decided there and then. Never again will I silence my own will, my knowledge from within and my dignity for someone to call themselves a specialist. Never again will I let anyone take my hope away from me and fill my mind with negative prospects. I slowly started walking towards the city centre. The steps were easy. The headache phased out with each breath. The jacket was unbuttoned at the neck and no longer sat too tight; the feeling of spring could circulate under the collar. I felt a smile spread across my reddish face. I thought of all the experts I have met over the years. It was a mixed crowd that gave me both good and less good experiences. Experiences of hope, despair, humiliation, insight, perspective and envy, but also of joy and confirmation. I thanked them all. Yes, in fact. Everyone had done their best based on their ability. Everyone had contributed to this moment of clarity, insight and inner freedom. I stopped and glanced back at the hospital window and all the life stories that hid behind the scenes. We never know where life will take us. I started walking again. Whatever happens in the future, I would at least enjoy

this very day that sparkled, gave me warmth and held me.